Palm Tree Of Life: All You Need To Know About Palm Fruit Oil

Palm Tree Of Life: All You Need To Know About Palm Fruit Oil

Jim Parker

Contents

About the Author

J. Parker believes that each choice you make regarding your food lifestyle acts as either a deposit or withdrawal in your "health banking" account. You can choose to make mostly savings deposits or check (cheque) withdrawals.

The balance of that account determines your energy, vitality, risk of disease, longevity and ultimately the quality of your life.

J. Parker has worked in big food companies creating concepts. J. Parker is also a pseudonym. J. Parker, fondly referred to as J.P, writes to inspire a healthy relationship with food and exercise, along with practical tips to incorporate healthy living.

Introduction: Palm Fruit Oil

Palm Fruit Oil is nature's gift. It has been in use for over 5000 years in Africa. It grows in the wild but recently it has been grown in large plantations in Malaysia and South East Asia.

This healthy tropical oil is derived from the fruit of the oil palm tree that grows in

Africa's jungles or the Malaysia's sustainable plantations. Palm oil is the world's first sustainable vegetable oil.

Palm fruit oil is a non-GMO oil and it is extremely versatile and has been enjoyed by billions of peoples for thousands of years. Palm fruit takes its color from beta-carotene, the precursor to vitamin A. It appears in three forms: retinol, retinal and retinoic acid.

Retinol enhances the body's defense system by bolstering the development of helper and natural killer cells, increasing the body's adaptive or acquired immunity.

The body's adaptive immunity helps in regenerating cells damaged by infection. For this purpose and others, the palm fruit oil is invaluable. It is a must have oil in your kitchen cabinet as it will save you many a doctor's visits.

Palm Tree of Life

Palm Fruit Oil Vs Palm Kernel Oil

Some say palm oil is bad for you. Some say it is good for you. What is the truth about this oil? The real issue is that many people do not have information for or against palm fruit oil supplementation (consumption). Where people have information, such information is sometimes convoluted.

While our African ancestors were getting busy supplementing their diets with red oil made from palm fruits, some scientists and medical authorities like W.H.O, were busy second-guessing whether or not palm fruit oil is good or bad for you.

They finally concluded that it is bad for you. That was not true then nor is it true today. It was like what was done with cholesterol before the real truth about LDL and HDL cholesterol were differentiated. We do not have to wait for such information any longer with regards to palm fruit oil.

Though, some of the medical authorities had thought that palmitic acid raised cholesterol levels if consumed, a 2002 Canadian study published in the "Asian Pacific Journal of Clinical Nutrition" examined the effects of high consumption of palmitic acid in humans and concluded that it does not raise cholesterol if it is combined with linoleic acid.

What?

But nature has done its science perfectly. The main ingredients in palm fruit oil includes palmitic, oleic and linoleic acids.

Palm fruit oil is 50 percent saturated fat and 50 percent unsaturated fat. It contains ~ 44% palmitic acid, 5% stearic acid, 39% oleic acid and 10% linoleic acid.

When palmitic acid was combined with lots of trans-fatty acids, LDL cholesterol levels rose and HDL cholesterol decreased. Nature has mixed many fine acids in good proportions to form Palm fruit oil.

As you can see, linoleic acid, an unsaturated fatty acid, is always found with palmitic acid in olive, palm and coconut oils. This means that palmitic acid is virtually never consumed apart from other healthier fats, so its negative impact on health might have been over-estimated previously. Highly over-estimated and bordering on outright lies.

Below are studies that show the many benefits and potentials of palm fruit oil. For the avoidance of any confusion palm fruit oil is not the same as palm oil.

 Palm fruit oil is derived from the fleshy part of the fruit while palm oil is derived from the kernel of the nut. Perhaps, it may be better to designate palm oil as palm kernel oil.

Palm kernel oil comes from the innermost kernel—nutlike core of the fruit. The kernel oil must not be confused with the fruit oil because it contains high amount of saturated fats. Studies show that highly saturated fats—kernel oil—are worse for you in diets than the dietary cholesterol that occurs in food.

Instead of using margarines and spreads with kernel oils,

you may want to replace those with tropical palm fruit oil.

There are quite a few tropical oils. They include palm fruit oil, coconut oil, palm kernel oil etc.

Palm Fruit Oil-------49% level of saturated fat
Coconut Oil---------92% level of saturated fat
Palm Kernel Oil----82% level of saturated fat

Palm Fruit oil is the best oil for your heart. Period!

It is natural. It is nature's fruit for a healthy heart. It is as natural as the Sun giving you vitamin D. A combination of the sunshine vitamin and the natural vitamin E and beta-carotene are the highway to a healthy heart.

You may be thinking right about now: What about Olive oil? Olive oil will be treated soon after the studies. Below are those studies that back up palm fruit oil consumption.

Palm Tree of Life

Studies that show more Benefits of Palm Fruit Oil

There are a series of studies from universities worldwide listing the many benefits and how-it-works of palm fruit oil.

You will be amazed at the benefits and you will wonder why this oil is not widely available in United States.

After reading these studies, I thought to myself: What

would the drug companies do if people knew all these benefits.

What would the companies that manufactures drugs for diabetes, cancer, immune, heart & cardiovascular issues, brain & cognitive issues and much more.

These studies are especially a must read for people suffering from any of the above listed conditions and much more.

1. On immune System & Cancer Benefits

In one study from University Putra, Malaysia, conducted by Mahalingam D., et al. (2011), it was observed that palm fruit tocols enhanced the immune response to vaccines. In the study, researchers showed that supplementing palm fruit tocotrienols of approximately—400mg per day—for 2 months, enhanced the immune response to a tetanus toxoid vaccination in humans who volunteered.

This therefore means that palm fruit tocotrienols can enhance the bodies' defense against pathological invasions.

Yet, in another study from Cancer Research Center, Malaysia, Nesaretnam, et al. (2010), it was observed that palm fruit tocols showed insignificant benefit in women with breast.

It was a human study that examined the effect of adding tocols
alongside tamoxifen therapy in women with breast cancer. Though
fewer participants died in the tocol group, the results were found to be non-significant because of the low number of study participants. A larger sample population for clinical trials are now under consideration.

In China's Harbin Medical University another study by

Xu WL., et al. (2009), palm fruit tocols was shown to inhibit the growth of human colon cancer cells.

This was a test tube study that showed inhibitory effects of palm fruit tocols on colon cancer cells. The tocotrienols had the strongest activity for inducing cancer cell death by increasing the Bax / Bcl-2 ratio, and activating caspase-3.

The Aga Khan University study led by Ashfaq MK, et al. (2000), palm fruit tocols & carotenoids is shown to increase natural killer cells. The study showed that palm fruit tocols and carotenoids enhanced natural killer cells, thereby strengthening the bodies' ability to fight and defeat foreign invaders.

The study showed that tocotrienols increased natural killer cells approximately 10x more effectively than regular vitamin E (alpha-tocopherol).

Another study from the University of Reading, England & Malaysia by Shah/Nesaretnam, et al. (1997-2006) showed that palm fruit tocols and carotenoids inhibit breast cancer growth through multiple mechanisms.

The studies explained the mechanism of action of tocols and carotenoids in breast cancer cells. The studies showed the suppression cancer through reduction of estrogen epoxidation, the activation of cancer cell death, and other non-ER mediated mechanisms. The findings suggest therapeutic benefits of palm fruit phytonutrients.

A study by Nesaretnam, et al. (1995) from Cancer Research Center, Ontario, showed that palm fruit tocols inhibit human breast cancer cells in the test tube.

Researchers found that palm fruit tocols inhibited growth

of breast cancer cells by at least 50% in test tubes. Meanwhile, regular vitamin E (alpha-tocopherol) had no effect.

These results tell us that a mixture of natural tocols from palm fruits (i.e., tocotrienols & tocopherols) have an effect over alpha-tocopherol alone. A study from the Research Center, France led by Nishino H, et al. (1989), found that palm fruit carotenoids suppressed human cancer cells in a test tube.

Researchers also found tumor suppressing effect in the stomach, skin, and pancreatic cancer cells from mixed carotenoids obtained from palm fruit oil.

One of the findings showed that the natural mixed carotenoids from palm fruit have a stronger tumor suppressing effect than a single carotenoid as in beta-carotene.

Palm Fruit Oil has been found to reduce breast cancer occurrence in rats. A study from the University of

Malaya conducted and led by Sundram K, et al. (1989) found that when Researchers administered cancer causing DMBA—DMBA is an immuno-suppressor and a powerful organ-specific laboratory carcinogen.

DMBA is widely used in researches studying cancer. DMBA serves as a tumor initiator—to rats whose diets were then enriched with red palm fruit oil. It was found that among other foods, diets with red palm fruit oil had the lowest incidence of cancer. This was because red palm oil naturally contains the highest concentration of oil soluble phytonutrients.

2. On Heart & Cardiovascular Benefits

Palm fruit tocols has been found to increase artery cleansing protein—APO-A1—in humans. A study from the Faculty of Medicine, Malaysia led by

Heng EC, et al. (2013) found that this study showed that palm fruit tocols increased APO-A1 by 73% after some month—six months or thereabout.

An increase in APO-A1 shows that palm fruit phytonutrients can enhance lipoprotein (HDL) quality and enhance the removal of plaque from blood vessel walls.

Palm fruit tocols improve and promote circulation by enhancing blood vessel blood flow. A study from the School of Medical Sciences, Malaysia led by Rasool AH, et al. (2008), found that the study after 6 weeks, participants had a 10% improvement in pulse wave velocity (blood vessel flexibility).

This means that palm fruit tocols can improve cardiovascular health by prolonging or increasing nitric oxide activity in the blood vessel wall.

In a study, there was this discovery of cholesterol lowering effect of tocotrienols in animals. A study from the University of Wisconsin authored by Qureshi, et al. (1986), also noted that researchers isolated and identified tocotrienols as the cholesterol lowering fraction from cereal grains.

This study found that tocotrienols lower LDL cholesterol at approximately 20% in fowls and quail. Palm fruit tocol extract being tocotrienols and tocopherols became the major focus in future research studies.

3. On Obesity & Diabetes

Discovery of cholesterol lowering effect of tocotrienols in animals was made in a study in University of Wisconsin by Qureshi, et al. (1986).

Researchers found that tocotrienols lower LDL cholesterol at (~20%) in chickens, quail, and swine. Palm fruit is extremely rich source of tocotrienols. Palm fruit tocol extract—tocotrienols & tocopherols) is a major focus for future research.

Today, 2/3 of Americans over the age of 20 are

obese. The story is the same in the UK. In UK, the government has considered declaring obesity a disability. The above statistics are very scary.

There are 7.1 million deaths worldwide resulting from heart disease. People are so fat; their organs are falling apart. A few years back 7.9 million deaths were due to cancer.

In a few years, it is estimated that cancer will claim 11million lives per year. In the year 2031, 336 million people worldwide will be diabetic.

However, palm fruit phytonutrients have been found to absorb into fat cells in Humans. After a collection of human studies by Ohio State University conducted by Wan Nazaimoon WM, et al. (2012), it was confirmed that consuming palm fruit phytonutrients through diet leads to increased tocols and carotenoids in fat tissue after 4-12 weeks.

A steady consumption of palm fruit oil provided evidence that these phytonutrients may reduce or prevent the formation of fat cells in humans.

Palm fruit tocols improve blood sugar control in diabetic mice. A study from Chinese Academy of Sciences, Fang F., et al. (2010), concluded that palm fruit tocols act as selective modulators of proliferator-activated receptors (PPARs) which increased insulin sensitivity and uptake of glucose by insulin responsive tissues.

Therefore, there was an improved glucose utilization. This suggests tocotrienols may help promote nutrient storage into muscle cells rather than fat cells.

Another study concluded that carotenoids inhibit fat cell formation in test-tube. The study done by Applied Life Sciences, Japan, by

Kawada T, et al. (2000), showed that carotenoids suppressed the growth of new fat cells by inhibiting PPAR-y2.

Additional researches discovered that palm fruit tocols encouraged fat cell death, suggesting that palm fruit carotenoids and tocols may have a synergistic effect against body fat.

4. On The Health of Your Liver

Palm fruit tocols is known to reduce liver stiffness in patients with non-alcoholic fatty liver disease. In a study from the Research Center, Philippines, Arguillas M., et al. (2013) showed that certain amount per day of palm fruit tocols reduced liver stiffness in approximately 8 out of 10 patients after a couple of months.

Palm fruit tocols was found to reverse liver damage in

many patients with end-stage liver disease. This was also a study from University of Ohio conducted by Sen CK., et al. (2012).

It was a study that was intended to identify the tissue distribution of tocotrienols after oral supplementation. The team observed that after providing the palm fruit tocotrienols, half of the patients no longer required liver transplants.

Due to this success, a stage II clinical trial to test palm

fruit extract for end-stage liver failure has been initiated. There are absolutely many benefits to ingesting palm fruit oil extracts.

Palm fruit tocols reverses non-alcoholic fatty liver disease. This was confirmed in a study from Universiti Sains Malaysia, Magosso E., et al. (2010). The study showed a reversal of non-alcoholic fatty liver disease (NAFLD) in approximately half of patients after approximately 12 months of supplementation with palm fruit tocols of daily. Researchers therefore theorized that NAFLD may be a result of a nutritional deficiency in tocotrienols. Palm fruit oil negates that deficiency.

5. On Brain & Cognitive Health

A University of Ohio study conducted by Sen CK., et al. (2012) established that palm fruit tocols has the ability to reach human brain tissue after oral supplementation.

Adding palm fruit oil to your meals like potato, soups, stew, porridge, beans is one sure way of supplementation.

The study established that dietary consumption of palm fruit tocols by ingesting palm fruit oils makes the tocols reach all vital organs in the body in about 3 months. Though more studies are needed here, available evidence found that clinically relevant concentrations of tocotrienols are found within the brain. This suggests that stroke benefits can be obtained in human tissue from oral supplementation of palm fruit oil.

Palm fruit tocols has been found to protect against glutamate induced cell death in rat brains. This University of California-Berkeley study by Sen CK., et al. (2000) showed the superiority of palm fruit tocols over a generic vitamin E—alpha-tocopherol—for neuroprotection from exposure to toxic levels of glutamate.

Such unexpected positive results have led to the study of palm fruit tocols for stroke protection in animals and ultimately humans.

Another conclusion from University of California-Berkeley by Sen CK., et al. (2011) was that palm fruit oil activated collateral blood supply after stroke event in dogs.

In the study, research made a group of dogs receive palm fruit tocols for 10 weeks while another group of dogs did not receive palm fruit tocols. The group that received the tocotrienols were protected from stroke due to an activation of small dormant vascular channels that feeds the brain with blood at a time when the primary artery was obstructed. The success was so positive that it led to development of human clinical studies.

Senescence:

Is a state of unnoticed aging, is a quality you can manage if you know how. It simply means you manage yourself nutritionally in such a way so that you live longer and healthy.

Senescence by definition means, growing old; aging but slowly. We can all assume that we all going to get old all things being equal. But how fast we get old becomes the issue.

When cells lose their ability to divide and replicate because of DNA damage or a shortening of telomeres, they go through a transformation called apoptosis—that is—they go through a decline— senescence—and/or a self-destruction result.

The ultimate end result of a cell is a cell death, which is a normal part of biological functioning. This occurs regularly in everyone's body.

One of the qualities of palm fruit is to prolong the cells of the body. Below are a series of studies pointing to that direction.

Skin & Anti-Aging Properties

Palm fruit tocols slow down the aging of skin. It does this so well by reducing advanced glycosylated end products (AGEs). A study from the Faculty of Medicine, Malaysia, Chin SF, et al. (2011) showed an approximate 39% reductions in the cross linking of glucose and proteins in grown adults after few months of palm fruit tocotrienol supplementation.

The findings show that palm fruit phytonutrients slow the aging process by reducing oxidative damage to structural proteins. When phytonutrient does this, it reduces or slows skin wrinkling and aging.

Still on aging, another study from University of Science, Malaysia by K.H. Yuen, et al. (2007) concluded that palm fruit tocols increase growth of scalp hairs in humans. The study showed an approximate 40%

increase in the number of scalp hairs in less than a year of palm fruit tocol diets. The # of hairs were increased in such thinning areas of the scalp for individuals suffering from hair loss.

Here is another study. Palm fruit phytonutrients accumulate into skin greater than other fat-soluble phytonutrients. This study is from the University of California-Berkeley by Weber, et al. (1997.

The study showed that palm fruit phytonutrients when supplemented, reach the skin tissue. The study showed that the palm fruit tocotrienols had a greater preference for skin tissue than other oil soluble phytonutrients—even—Vitamins A, Vitamin E, and CoQ-10.

Palm fruit tocols even provided better protection against sun rays damage.

The way you may see it is, that you may have to learn to adapt to new tastes, so as to acquire a route to better health. If you really want to understand the effect of phytonutrients on the skin, stop an African who you know uses palm fruit oil and ask what their age is. You'd be shocked.

What are a few disturbances to your usual tastes when your health and longevity is at stake?

The biggest problem in understanding this oil is the interchange of words. Palm oil is interchangeably used for palm fruit oil and palm kernel oil. Palm Fruit oil is very different from Palm kernel oil based on their composition.

Palm Fruit Oil is not palm oil. Palm Fruit oil is traditionally made mostly in Africa and Asia. It is made to maintain the natural nutrients of carotenes—the precursors to Vitamin A—

and is the antioxidant tocotrienols aka Vitamin E.

Tropically germinating in the wild, typically refined, bleached and deodorized, palm oil fruits have some fibers stripped from them resulting in a clear oil.
In its natural state, palm oil is red in color. Very red. This is due to a high concentration of carotenes and tocols. This is nature's style of providing protection for your heart.
Carotenes usually, are hydrocarbons found in

orange, yellow, and red vegetables. Such includes beta and alpha carotene and lycopene. For some understanding, a definition of some terms need be explained.

Beta Carotene and other Pro-Vitamin A carotenoids are alpha-carotene, and beta-cryptoxanthin that are converted into vitamin A or retinol. Retinol is the active form of vitamin A in the body.

Retinol are found in many yellow fruits and vegetables. Beta carotene is perhaps the most widely studied carotenoid ever.

Meanwhile, lycopene is responsible for the red color in fruits and vegetables like watermelon, tomatoes, red grapes, pink grapefruit etc.

Lycopene is also found in papayas and apricots. Though, it does not convert to vitamin A, it may have important cancer fighting properties and some other health benefits too.

The benefits of most carotenes like those in corn, tomatoes, and carrots etc., is enhanced by cooking them, especially in oil like palm fruit oil, olive, canola, or another monounsaturated oil.

Cooking can also destroy certain nutrients, such as vitamin C, in these vegetables. Cooking can also reduce the benefits in olive oil. Palm fruit oil can withstand heat better than some other oils.

Palm fruit oil comes from a tropical palm tree—elaeis guineensis—which is native to the tropical areas of Africa. It especially abundant in the West African areas of Africa where it grows in the wild.

Palm Fruit oil is a traditional oil used in Africa for more than 5000 years. In some localities there are small-scale family farms but mostly the trees grow in the wild. It was from Africa that the palm tree was introduced to Malaysia and South East Asia in the early 1900s. Malaysia is now the world leader in exports of palm oil. In Malaysia they are usually grown in large farms.

Other oils and fats generally are susceptible to attack by atmospheric oxygen, resulting in rancidity. Palm fruit oil contains tocols (Vitamin E) which are powerful natural antioxidants.

It, therefore, has exceptional resistance to rancidity. Palm fruit oil is known for its excellent stability at high temperatures thus it retains its benefits at such temperatures unlike many other oils.

Vitamin E - The Tocotrienols as Super Antioxidants

Vitamin E is one of the most important phytonutrients you find in palm fruit oil. It consists of eight naturally occurring isomers, a family of four tocopherols—alpha, beta, gamma and delta— and four tocotrienols—alpha, beta, gamma and delta—homologues.

There are mostly Vitamin E supplements on the market today which are composed of the more common tocopherols. Tocotrienols are believed to be a much more potent antioxidant than tocopherols.

Tocotrienols are naturally present in most plants. They are however, found mostly abundant in palm fruit oil extracted from palm fruits.

There are other sources such as rice, wheat germ, oat and barley.
Many published studies show that alpha-tocotrienol is more potent than alpha-tocopherol as a form of Vitamin E. Since tocotrienols are a form of Vitamin E found less abundantly in nature than tocopherols, the research on this super antioxidant is still recent and ongoing.

It will not be surprising if tocotrienols becomes

recognized and consumed as the new super antioxidant in the very near future. Palm fruit oil is one of your best sources for Vitamin E. Most Vitamin E supplements and skin care products on the market today are soy-based.

Nature has provided us with almost 600 known carotenoids, ranging from yellow orange to red hues and some of these possess Vitamin A activity of varying degrees. Palm fruit oil is one of the richest natural plant sources of carotenoids with concentration in the range of 500–700 parts per million—ppm.

Palm fruit oil has over 15 times more carotenoids than carrots and 300 times more than tomatoes. What differentiates Palm fruit oil from others is the quantity of its carotenoids. No other vegetable oil contains carotenoids in such significant quantities like palm fruit oil. Analysis shows that alpha and beta carotenes constitute approximately 90% of the total carotenoid content.

Carotenoids are organic pigments that are found in the chloroplasts and chromoplasts of plants and some other photosynthetic organisms. Carotenoids, the colorful plant pigments some of which the body can turn into vitamin A, are powerful antioxidants that can help prevent some forms of cancer and heart disease, and act to enhance your immune response to infections.

These precursors to vitamin A are sometimes called provitamin A. Bright-orange beta-carotene is the most important carotenoid for adequate vitamin A intake because it yields more vitamin A than alpha-carotene or gamma-carotene.

The odds are that you consume palm oil/palm kernel products frequently — you just don't know it. In Africa and Asia, where the vast majority of palm fruit oil is produced and consumed, it is a common cooking oil. Here in the U.S., it's estimated that palm oil products or ingredients derived from it are used in a lot of the products on the average supermarket shelf.

Let us check out a few of the products that you may find palm oil ingredients. It's in your cookies, your baked goods, your margarines, your lipsticks and skin lotions.

Others are your shampoo, your various kinds of toothpastes and a wide range of other packaged foods and personal care products like soaps.

This is due to, in part, that palm oil is a highly versatile product that lends itself well to food products and processing.

Palm fruit oil is naturally free of trans fats. That makes it a very good oil but you must be able to know the difference between palm fruit oil and palm kernel oil. Both oils come from the same tree but are totally different.

One is very good for your heart and the other is not so good. Palm Fruit oil is enriched with vitamin E and beta-carotene. Palm fruit is oil-rich with reddish-black skin and yellow-orange fleshy part.

It comes from the red palm tree, or Elaeis guineensis. Elaeis guineensis is the species of palm commonly called palm fruit oil or macaw-fat. It is the principal source of palm fruit oil and palm kernel oil.

It is native to west and southwest Africa, specifically the area between Angola and the Gambia. The species name guineensis refers to the name for the area—Guinea--and not the modern country which bears that name today.

A native of Africa, the fruit has been used in oil

production for centuries over centuries. Flavorful, nutritious and healthy, palm fruit oil is one of the most natural sources of beta-carotene and vitamin E.

Palm fruit oil comes from the fleshy, orange part of the fruit, and is rich in monounsaturated or "good" fats. Palm fruit oil is an important part of an oil blend that can support healthy cholesterol levels already within the normal range. Palm kernel oil, on the other hand, comes from the innermost kernel, or nut-like core, of the plant.

The kernel contains highly saturated fats that can clog arteries. Studies indicate that highly saturated fats like palm kernel oils are worse for you than the dietary cholesterol that occurs in foods.

This suggests that instead of eating margarines or spreads with palm kernel oil, use great-tasting, creamy-red palm fruit oil.

While palm fruit and Canola oils are trending among both health-conscious choosers and gourmet cooks, there is still some confusion about where and when to use this healthy oil versus olive oil and others.

There are factors that should be considered. These factors include your current cholesterol level and the temperature needed to prepare your desired dish.

Cooking Temperature Considerations

Every cooking oil has a temperature benchmark called a smoke point. This is the temperature at which is the heated oil causes both the taste and the nutrient level to breakdown.

The oil can actually become toxic if it is heated well beyond its smoke point.

Otherwise toxic fumes can be created from oil that is overheated. There are oils with smoke points that can stand higher temperatures and they still add flavor to the food that makes it even more delicious.

Cooking at temperatures higher than an oil's smoke point can damage some oils. Unless an oil is suitable, high heat may cause your food to taste bitter or scorched.

The layman's easiest way to read and know whether the oil has reached its smoke point is when the oil starts to yield thick smoke. If the heat is not turned down, the oil is likely to flame up. People inhale this smoke every day.

Perhaps, they think it's healthy, but in reality, the smoke from heated olive oil is full of toxins. Olive oil is better off used as is—room temperature—or at very low temperatures of below 250 degrees.

Some smoke points for different oils:

Olive oil should be heated below 250 degrees. Depending on the type, olive oil can have a smoke point of up to 468F

Smoke point: Olive oil— smoke point ranges from 320—468F depending on the type of olive oil: Extra Virgin is 320°F, Virgin is

420°F, Pomace is 460°F, Extra Light is 468°F

Grape seed oil
Smoke point – at least 400 degrees

Coconut oil
Smoke point – 350 degrees

Canola Oil
Smoke point—450F

Macadamia Nut oil
Smoke point – approximately 413 degrees

Palm Fruit Oil

Smoke point—
approximately 425 degrees

Prepping the Palm Fruits

There are various ways you can prep to eat the palm fruits.

1. You may pick a few of the seeds that fell from the palm and chew on it raw after washing just like snacks

2. You may cook a few of the fruits for about 30mins. Drain the hot water and sprinkle with a pinch of salt for an evening snack.

3. Soups/porridge: You may want to boil a plateful of palm fruits (50-100) for 30 minutes. Drain the hot water and leave to cool from hot to warm. Transfer to a bigger/wider bowl where the seeds are then squished with the palms. The intent is to

squeeze and filter the fleshy part from the nuts.

After squeezing and squishing, you would notice when the paste is very thick. Add some water, mix properly and filter the liquids onto the pot you intend to cook soup or porridge with. You can now add your ingredients as when cooking with regular oil.

The oil in the extract will float to the top of your soup when your food is done/cooked. The palm fruit extract used in cooking any soup/porridge/stew is a little different from the palm fruit oil.

Palm fruit oil is pure oil extracted from the palm fruit pulp while the palm fruit extract described here is unprocessed and is as natural as it gets. This extract even contains less saturated fat than palm fruit oils.

Where Can I Buy Palm Fruit Oil?

If you live in the West in cities like

New York,

Chicago,

Long Island,

Newark, NJ,

London,

Brussels,

Frankfurt or Amsterdam,

You can buy palm fruit oil from African grocery stores known as African Markets. Now, you can also buy this oil at Walmart. Some Caribbean grocery stores have this product on the shelf. You can also get them in Malaysian/Asian grocery stores located in such large cities listed above.

They come in many names but be careful to ask for palm fruit oil. Some labels may have palm fruit oil as red palm oil. They are usually the same. You just have to be aware that palm fruit oil is not the same as palm kernel oil.

Comparing Palm Fruit Oil and Olive Oil

Palm oil is 50 percent saturated fat and 50 percent unsaturated fat. It contains ~ 44% palmitic acid, 5% stearic acid, 39% oleic acid—Oleic acid is a monounsaturated fatty acid found naturally in many plant sources and animal products.

It is an omega-9 fatty acid, and is considered one of the healthier sources of fat in the diet. Some health experts recommend using it in cooking and a number of so-called health foods and diet products will use this compound in place of animal fats.

Palm fruit oil also contains 10% linoleic acid (polyunsaturated).

Linoleic acid is a polyunsaturated fatty acid and is one of two fatty acids that we cannot produce but must be obtained from food sources. Linoleic acid is a type of fat, or fatty acid, found in Palm fruit and vegetable oils, nuts, seeds and animal products.

An essential omega-6 fatty acid, linoleic acid is required by the human body in small amounts. Too much, however, can be detrimental to your health.

Consumers of a standard American diet are much more likely to get too much linoleic acid than too little. But with the right balance, saturated fatty acids maintain your HDL—the good cholesterol—while polyunsaturated fatty acids decrease your LDL—the bad cholesterol.

Therefore, if your cholesterol is elevated, choose an oil rich in polyunsaturates, or even one of the more liquid fractions of palm fruit oil which contains a healthy balance of polyunsaturated and saturated fatty acids as well as antioxidant-rich carotenoids and vitamin E.

Palm fruit oil is a very good mix for elevated cholesterol level. It helps you stabilize your cholesterol to optimum levels.

Olive oil contains 72 percent monounsaturated fat, 14 percent saturated fat and 9 percent polyunsaturated fat. Olive oil is very good for you if your cholesterol level is normal.

This is because Olive oil is mostly monounsaturated fatty acids. If your cholesterol is in the healthy range, consuming olive oil is fine and won't negate it since monounsaturated fatty acids are neutral.

Though olive oil won't cause trouble with your cholesterol it cannot get you out of trouble if your body is desperately needing more polyunsaturated fatty acids.

What you must draw from this is that you must know your cholesterol levels at all times and thus choose the needed oil for supplementation.

A blanket sales pitch like "this oil is the best" that you hear so often is always not true. The best oil for Janet might not be the best oil for John.

In fact, the oil that is good for John in January might not be good for him in

December because his cholesterol levels may have just changed.

As you read through the comparison above pay special attention to saturated fatty acids and polyunsaturated fatty acids. Understanding your cholesterol range could help you decide which oil is best for you.

Palm fruit oil can be a heart-healthy choice when consumed as part of a balanced diet. It has been consumed in Africa for centuries and in Asia for almost a century.

No oil is good for your heart when used in large quantities; in moderation, however, palm fruit oil delivers a balance of fats and some of the antioxidants needed to maintain a healthy heart.

Antioxidants are substances or nutrients in our foods which can prevent or slow the oxidative damage to our body. When our body cells use oxygen, they naturally produce free radicals—by-products—that can cause serious damages.

Antioxidants act as "free radical scavengers" and hence prevent and repair damage done by these free radicals. Health problems such as heart disease, macular degeneration, diabetes, cancer are all contributed by oxidative damage.

Antioxidants may also enhance immune defense

and therefore lower the risk of cancer and infection. If you think about it, we eat a whole lot of oils in our diet. Almost every food is cooked or garnished with some kind of oil or fat.

 With that information in hand, rather than choose the "best" oils with or without a high content of polyunsaturated or a lower content of saturated fatty acids would not be the issue but when to eat higher saturated/polyunsaturated

and or
saturated/monounsaturated.

The Benefits of eating Palm Fruit Oil

When you cook with palm fruit oil, it helps your systems.

Palm Fruit Oil Boosts the Immune Function

Palm fruit color comes from beta-carotene—the precursor of vitamin A which are in three forms: retinol, retinal and retinoic acid.

Retinol enhances the body's defense system. It does this through bolstering the development of helper and natural killer cells thereby increasing the body's adaptive and/or acquired immunity and regenerating cells that were damaged by infections.

 The immune system is typically divided into two categories–innate and adaptive–although these distinctions are not mutually exclusive.

The adaptive immune or specific immune response consists of antibody responses and cell-mediated responses, which are carried out by different lymphocyte cells, B cells and T cells, respectively. Our adaptive immune system saves us from certain death by infection. An infant born with a severely defective adaptive immune system will most likely die unless extraordinary measures are taken to isolate it from a host of infectious diseases.

Adaptive immunity is, therefore, a process where immune cells learn to improve defenses by memory. There is a study published in a 1992 issue of the *Journal of Pediatrics* where it was reported that 10 of the 20 children with measles were vitamin A-deficient.

Remember that palm fruit oil is a reservoir of beta-carotene. Measles as a highly contagious viral infection producing various symptoms and a rash can easily kill a child lacking in Vitamin A.

Palm Fruit Oil Helps Fight Cancer

Tocotrienols which is the lesser-known form of biologically active vitamin E, are powerful antioxidants and anti-cancer agents. Palm fruit oil contains a lot of tocotrienol. Palm fruit oil contains above 40 percent gamma tocotrienol. A study published in a 2008 issue of the *British Journal of*

Cancer found that gamma tocotrienol starts the preliminary drive to killing prostate cancer cells. It's the beginning of apoptosis.

In another study published in a 2010 issue of *Journal of Nutritional Biochemistry,* researchers found that tocotrienol decreases spread and or the invasion in the first place of human gastric cancer cells by reducing the development of certain enzymes which limits the suppression (death) of cancer cells.

Helps Protect Brain Cells

Alpha tocotrienol which is a potent antioxidant, makes up 20 percent of the natural vitamin E in palm fruit oil. In a study published in the 2010 issue of the *Journal of the American College of Nutrition* found that alpha tocotrienol prevented the oxidation of arachidonic acid.

Arachidonic acid, the most abundant polyunsaturated fatty acid in the central nervous system, is vulnerable to oxidation under stress such as ischemic stroke, when blood supply to the brain is temporarily insufficient.

Palm Fruit Oil Helps Fight Night Blindness

Night blindness (also called nyctalopia) is the inability to see well at night or in poor light. It is not a disease, but rather a symptom of an underlying disorder or problem, especially untreated nearsightedness. Though there are many causes of night blindness, Vitamin A deficiency is a likely suspect.

Palm fruit is abundant with beta-carotene that can be easily converted to retinal in the body. Retinal helps to fight night blindness. When light passes through the cornea, it lands on the cells of the retina and rhodopsin reacts.

As this happens the retinal changes its configuration

and separates from opsin. This leads to the destruction of some retinal. By diet supplementation of palm fruit oil, vitamin A can easily be replenished.

Palm Fruit Oil Helps Protect the Heart functions

In one review published in a 2001 issue of *Experimental*

Biology and Medicine researchers noted that alpha-tocopherol in palm fruit oil prevents the oxidation of LDL cholesterol. It also reduces platelet aggregation. It also enhances blood vessel dilation. All the above makes for an efficient blood flow.

The Conclusion

With all these studies and all these benefits, you start to wonder why palm fruit oil is not readily available in the American markets. You would think that with so much benefits coming from the use of palm fruit oil, the American market would be saturated with the product.

Perhaps, there have not been sufficient information.

The health benefits of olive oil have been touted for many of years.

At a point, coconut oil become all the rage and hailed by many as the king of oils. Whatever oil is in your kitchen cabinet—whether olive, coconut, groundnut, almond, canola, safflower, walnut, or avocado oils – none compares to the powerful nutritional virtues of organic palm fruit oil.

The health benefits of palm fruit oil can be achieved by incorporating only 2 to 4 tablespoons into your soups and stew, jollof rice, beans etc. Palm fruit oil is especially good for frying.

That the Egyptian and other civilizations have used palm fruit oil for centuries attest to palm fruit oil being one of the most nutritious and beneficial edible oil in the world today.

The inability for so long to distinguish the benefits of

other products from the palm tree from palm fruit oil is perhaps why the palm fruit is not known in more households as it should be.

The stigma attached to the *palm kernel oil* has kept the palm fruit oil in the dark. When it comes to oils palm fruit oil is otherwise a bona fide food.

Palm fruit oil has a powerhouse of antioxidant nutrients. The same ones that give tomatoes, carrots, some other fruits and vegetables their rich red and orange colors.

Palm fruit oil contains more antioxidants than tomatoes or carrots. Red palm fruit oil is also densely packed with tocotrienols—a powerful form of vitamin E.

If you do not have a bottle at home, now is the time to write it down in your things to purchase list because Palm fruit oil is it.

Palm Tree of Life

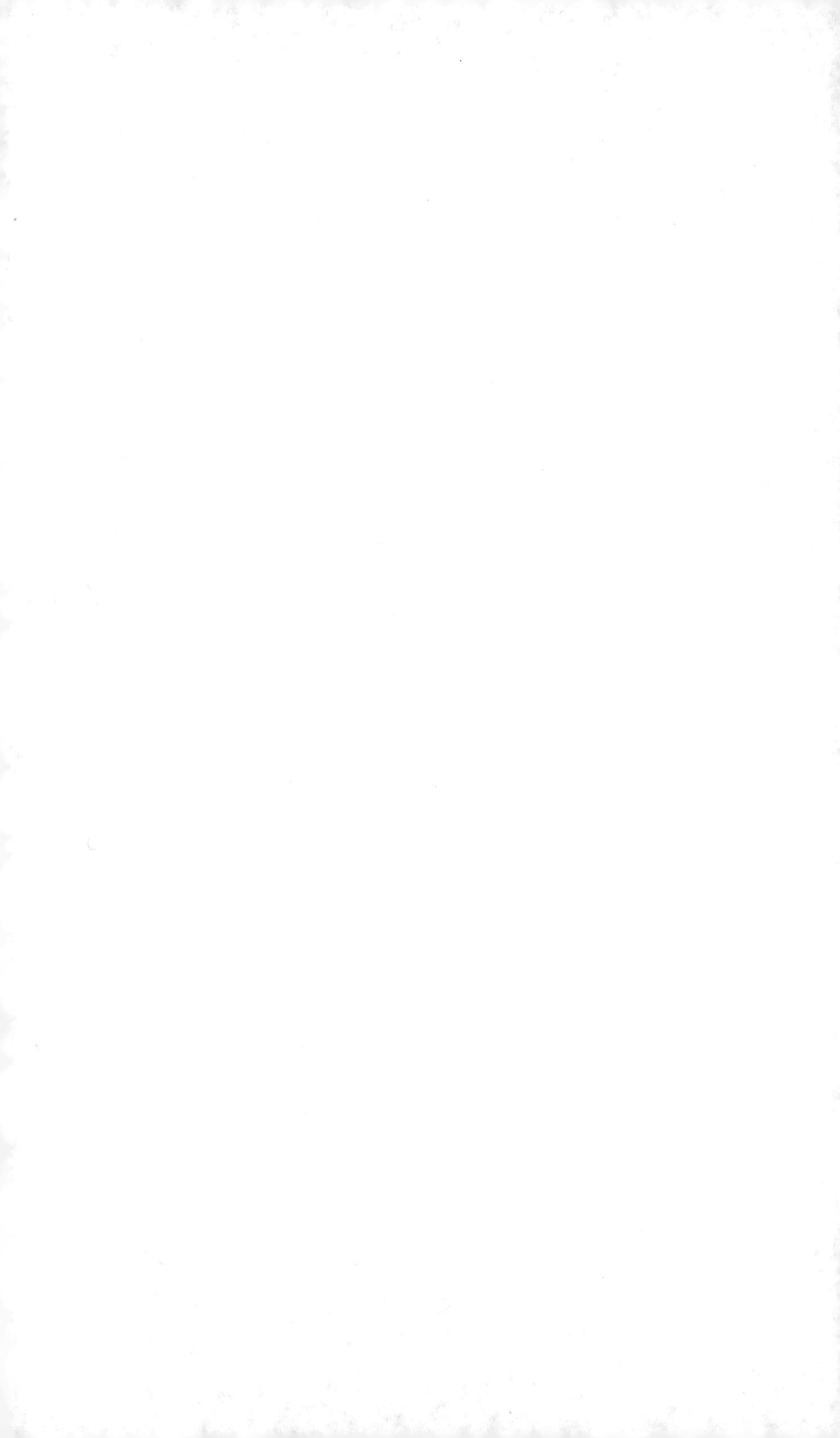